100 Foods That Heal Your Body

100 Foods That Heal Your Body

Alfred E. Dawson

Writers Club Press

San Jose New York Lincoln Shanghai

100 Foods That Heal Your Body

Writers Club Press
an imprint of iUniverse.com, Inc.

For information address:
iUniverse.com, Inc.
620 North 48th Street, Suite 201
Lincoln, NE   68504-3467
www.iuniverse.com

ISBN: 0-595-14438-1

Printed in the United States of America

One of the leading causes of death in America is heart disease. Eating the proper foods on a daily basis, can greatly reduce your chances of heart disease.

Contents

Why Foods Heal Your Body xi

Introduction xiii

1 Apples 1

2 Apricots 2

3 Asparagus 3

4 Avocado 4

5 Bananas 5

6 Bass (fish) 6

7 Beans 7

8 Beets 8

9 Berries 9

10 Brazil Nuts 10

11 Bread (wheat) 11

12 Broccoli 12

13 Brussels sprouts 13

14 Buttermilk 14

15 Cabbage 15

16 Cantaloupe (melon) 16

17 Carrots 17

18 Cashew Nuts 18

19 Cauliflower 19

20 Celery 20

21 Cereal 21

22 Cherries 22

23 Chicken (poultry) 23

24 Chives 24

25 Clams 25

26 Coconut 26

27 Cod (fish) 27

28 Corn 28

29 Cottage Cheese 29

30 Cranberries 30

31 Cucumbers 31

32 Dates 32

33 Eggplant 33

34 Fish 34

35 Fruit 35

36 Grapes 36

37 Garlic 37

38 Grapefruit 38

39 Greens 39

40 Haddock (fish) 40

41 Herbs 41

42 Honey 42

43 Honeydew (melon) 43

44 Juice 44

45 Ketchup 45

46 Kiwifruit 46

47 Lamb 47

48 Lemons 48

49 Lettuce 49

50 Limes 50

51 Lobster 51

52 Mangoes 52

53 Milk 53

54 Mushrooms 54

55 Oatmeal 55

56 Okra 56

57 Olives 57

58 Onions 58

59 Oranges 59

60 Parsley 60

61 Pasta 61

62 Peaches 62

63 Peas 63

64 Pears 64

65 Pecan 65

66 Peppers (green) 66

67 Peppers (red) 67

68 Perch (fish) 68

69 Pineapples 69

70 Plums 70

71 Pollack (fish) 71

72 Pomegranates 72

73 Potatoes (Irish) 73

74 Poultry 74

75 Prunes 75

76 Pumpkins 76

77 Radishes 77

78 Raisins 78

79 Rice 79

80 Salmon (fish) 80

81 Sardines 81

82 Soups 82

83 Soybeans 83

84 Spinach 84

85 Sprouts 85

86 Squash 86

87 Strawberries 87

88 Tangerines 88

89 Tofu 89

90 Tomatoes 90

91 Trout 91
92 Tuna 92
93 Turnips 93
94 Vegetables 94
95 Walnuts 95
96 Watermelons 96
97 Wheat Germ 97
98 Yams (sweet potato) 98
99 Yeast (brewers) 99
100 Yogurt 100
A Gram of Prevention 101
The Body's Organs 102
What Minerals and Vitamins Really Do For The Body 104
Food Sources For Minerals and Vitamins 106
Protein 112
Vitamin B-Complex 113
Amino Acid 114
Antioxidants 116
Fiber 117
The Sweet Tooth 118
Water 120
Sunlight 121
Exercise 122
Afterthought 123
About the Author 125
Sources 127

Why Foods Heal Your Body

The body uses nutrients from minerals and vitamins to restore the cells and tissues while keeping the body's vital organs, such as the heart, the kidneys, the liver and lungs free from infections.

Natural foods do contain antioxidants, (something like a cleanser) that fight infections, bad bacteria and help prevent diseases. Keeping the body clean inside is part of what *natural foods* do.

When you know what is good for your body and you do it, it improves your health, prolong your life and makes you happy in more ways that you can measure.

In addition, natural foods help provide the lost energy sources, needed for normal health. When these lost minerals and vitamins restore the body's energy level, and provide the nutrition your body needs, either from a loss that is caused by injury or age, your body is being healed.

Introduction

Foods that heal the body provide the essential ingredients, that includes the minerals and vitamins, offering the nutrients that are an absolute necessity for the body to maintain good health.

Nutrients—Nutrients coincide with the word nutrition. Nutrients makeup the substance that provide nutrition, which is nourishment for the body. Nutrients that are essential for the human body includes: minerals, vitamins, carbohydrates and fats.

Minerals—Minerals from foods includes: calcium, chlorine, chromium, iodine, iron, magnesium, manganese, phosphorus, potassium, selenium, sodium and zinc.

Vitamins—Vitamins are commonly known by the letters A, B, C, D and E. Vitamins also include a variety of types, such as the B-Complex, known by numbered B's, such as B-1 or B-12. All of these vitamins are essential to excellent health.

The body receives *carbohydrates* and *fats* through the normal intake of protein.

1

Apples

Minerals: Magnesium, Silicon, Sodium
Vitamins: A

Apples are a great snack. The antioxidants the body receives, can neutralize the molecules that float in the main blood stream. Apples help the body eliminate the molecules that float in the main bloodstream, generally those molecules that contribute to heart disease.

Apples also help prevent cancer. Apples do contain flavonoids, another antioxidant that can fight-off infections. These flavonoids also help clean the arteries to keep them from clogging. Apples contain fiber. Very high in fiber, apples contain more fiber than wheat bread and cereal, which are know to be great foods in the reduction of the blood cholesterol level.

2

Apricots

Minerals: Calcium
Vitamins: A, C

The apricot is a fruit. There are a wide variety of apricots. Most of them resemble the peach, but are somewhat smaller. The apricot has a very delicate flavor when fresh. Many uses include the making of jam, canning and even fried for packaging.

The importance of the natural vitamins received through fruits can not be overlooked when it comes to the apricot.   A source of vitamins A and C, the apricot can often be an option for fruit, for those that do not like the taste of other fruits.

Also a source of calcium and phosphorus in its natural state, many fruits offer an acid to the body that help prevent internal diseases, easily developed when the body remains extremely low on bacteria fighting agents.

3

Asparagus

Minerals: Silicon, Iodine
Vitamins: A, C

The ascorbic acid that is provided from asparagus to the human body, gives the body an agent that will fight heart disease and cancer.

Asparagus is a very healthy food for the human body. Providing different minerals to give the body needed protection against unwanted infections, asparagus is a good source of needed vitamins.

Foods do heal the body and asparagus will do that as a natural green food. Asparagus is an herb. Originally grown in fresh sandy soil, it takes more that a year for the asparagus to fully develop to be cultivated.

Asparagus can also be grown indoors, like a normal house plant.

4

Avocado

Minerals: Iron, Phosphorus, calcium
Vitamins: A

The body depends on iron for a source of oxygen through food. Iron improves the red blood cells in the body. An anemic suffers from a shortage of iron in their body. A shortage of iron causes many ailments to the body which includes: fatigue, dry hair, pale skin and mental slowness.

Avocado is a fruit. As a good source of protein for the human body, avocado is known for it's nutty flavor.

The flavor and taste of many foods is what causes some people to like them. In a number of cases, there are foods that do not have a distinct taste to admire. When other foods do not have an attractive flavor or distinct taste, usually, natural foods can be used to enhance or even provide a good taste. Foods that provide juice and seasoning can often give non-tasting foods an added flavor and a reason to enjoy them.

5

Bananas

Minerals: Potassium, calcium, phosphorus
Vitamins: A

The banana is another one of the most nourishing foods for the body. Full of potassium, this food will nourish the body's cells.

Without the potassium our body generally needs, a variety of ailments and conditions can harm the body. Everything from poor heart beats to the inability to sleep properly, can result from a lack of potassium.

Fruit is the most nourishing food for the human body. Needed on a daily basis as the daily routine of activities take place, the body absorbs the intake that is stored inside. It is imperative that fruits of a variety are always included in daily menus for the body to receive it's supply of nutrients.

It is not uncommon to eat fruit more that three times a day to obtain the required minerals, vitamins and total nutrients to keep the body healthy.

6

Bass (fish)

Minerals: Protein, Phosphorus
Vitamins: A, E

A good reason to eat fish is to receive the cod-liver oil and the high source of protein that fish gives the body.

Vitamin E is one of the miracles for the human body. Everything from prolonging youth, to preventing sickness, this is the area where life gets prolonged due to good nutritious values found in what is rarely offered in other foods, cod-liver oil. Cod-liver oil contribute to the longevity of the body's cells life.

An anti-oxidant for the body, which is a detoxifying agent that help destroy fat inside the body, vitamin E can do wonders toward improving your health.

Fish is one of the healthy sources of protein for the body.

7

Beans

Minerals: Phosphorus, calcium, iron
Vitamins: A, B-6 (Pyridoxine)

High in fiber and protein, beans are one of the most nutritious foods for the body. There are a variety of beans: green beans; lima beans; kidney beans or any other bean, provides sources of nutrients the body needs. As a healthy choice for the body, few can match the life source of the bean. The most common edible beans have always been popular throughout the world.

Navy beans can be one of the more popular type due to their ease to digest. A natural food, beans give the body rewarding nutrition.

A source of potassium too, the bean can be a real life saver. The Vitamin B-6 is good for the nerves, muscles and the skin, often found in beans. A lack of Vitamin B-6 in the body can lead to many ailments, such as depression or even clogged arteries. Vitamin B-6, known as pyridoxine, an amino acid, helps the body destroy cancer causing agents.

8

Beets

Minerals: Sodium, Iron, Calcium, Phosphorus
Vitamins: A

Beets are a healer for the body. Helping lower blood pressure while improving your blood circulation, beets can also aid in cleaning the blood .

Few foods can combine the healing minerals beets can provide the human body. Beets contain a juice that provides what is needed for the kidneys and the liver. Maintaining a healthy body begins with foods that destroy unwanted excess inside the arteries, veins, blood vessels, the bladder and the colon. The parts of the body that are prone to disease or failure, are the ones that deserve the highest degree of therapeutic foods.

The mineral *sodium* which is salt, is an absolute necessity for the body and is found in most foods. A natural source of sodium is less harmful to the body than refined salt.

9

Berries

Minerals: Calcium, Phosphorus
Vitamins: A, C

Raspberries come in red, blue and black. Blackberries are higher in calcium that blueberries. Raspberries are fruits that can be grown in the home garden. The canning of raspberries is a very common practice.

As a natural food, the raspberry can provide a necessary nutrient the body needs for normal development. The prevention of diseases inside the body is due to the amount of antioxidants that is contained in the body.

Vitamin C is one of the primary protection mechanisms in the prevention of cancer and heart disease. High concentrations of Vitamins A and C inside the body help repair damaged tissues as well as help lower blood cholesterol levels.

Natural sources of the Vitamins A and C combined in fruits such as berries, can help eliminate deficiencies of these vitamins within the body.

10

Brazil Nuts

Minerals: Calcium, Phosphorus
Vitamins: A

Brazil nuts are a natural fruit that provides the body with nutrition in a variety of ways. Nuts can often be eaten as a snack, while there is an intake of essential minerals and an antioxidant, Vitamin A.

Many of the body's ailments and diseases are directly related to the lack of minerals and vitamins that fight infections and bad bacterial that leads to cancer.

When the body is protected with its needed supply of minerals and vitamins, which can easily be obtained through the eating of natural fruits and vegetables, the risk remains very low, that some type of disease will develop.

The brazil nut is one of the variety of sources that can be used to help provide the needed nutrition the body uses from Vitamin A, calcium and phosphorus, which play a vital role in preventing many ailments.

11

Bread (wheat)

Minerals: Phosphorus, Calcium
Vitamins: B-Complex, Niacin

There are two distinct breads that are good for the body—wheat and rye bread. Whole wheat bread provides the body with needed calcium and phosphorus.

Bread has always been a source of nutrition. Some breads are more nutritious than others. Wheat and rye bread gives the body additional minerals needed for good health.

Bread has always been a part of regular meals. The process in making bread includes the use of yeast. Yeast is needed as an element to heal the body. When added with flour and including rye or wheat, the bread becomes extremely healthy. Generally, baking your own bread can provide a source of excellent nutrition.

12

Broccoli

Minerals: Calcium, Phosphorus
Vitamins: A

Most people hate broccoli, but the human body loves it. One of the highest sources of Vitamin A when raw, broccoli is definitely a healing food for the human body.

Vitamin A can be overlooked sometimes for its importance to the body. Our vision, in which the eyes must focus repeatedly, requires a healthy amount of Vitamin A. Our skin and hair depends on the quantity of Vitamin A that the body receives. One part of the body that is protected by Vitamin A is the mucus membrane. It is the health of the mucus membrane that determines sinus conditions, hay fever, and allergies.

More important than any, the antioxidant in broccoli help prevent the development of lung cancer.

The fatigue we experience, is often a lack of Vitamin A in the body.

13

Brussels sprouts

Minerals: Phosphorus, Calcium
Vitamin: A, B, C

Brussels sprouts is a vegetable that resemble the cabbage. The leafy greens that are cooked in brussels sprouts are a healthy edible garden plant that deserves inclusion in meals, due to their multiple nutritious value in Vitamins A, B and C.

Vitamins are one of the ultimate protectors of the human body against cancer. Vitamin A as well as Vitamin C, can give the body a wealth of needed antioxidants that prevent the development of infections and spread of bacteria, that is unwanted, inside the body.

The B-Vitamins, come in a number of types. The B-Complex itself is what provide good metabolism. B Vitamins help promote the body's energy source.

14

Buttermilk

Minerals: Calcium, Phosphorus
Vitamins: A

Yes buttermilk is healthy. Buttermilk is a by-product of whole milk. Buttermilk is often overlooked as a healthy food for the body. When you are unsure if you have received all your body's needs in vitamins and minerals, then drink a small amount of buttermilk.

Buttermilk provides a list of minerals that include: potassium, sodium, chlorine, phosphorus, calcium, proteins and sulfur. All of these are needed by the body for restoring your health and healing the body.

The body also needs casein, which is found in buttermilk. The bacteria that contained in buttermilk is necessary to help replace the healthy bacteria the body looses from day to day. The acidity in buttermilk is also an agent will help prevent a variety of diseases and infections.

15

Cabbage

Minerals: Phosphorus, Calcium
Vitamins: A

Cabbage is a green leafy vegetable that is healthy for the body. Cabbage is considered a herb. As you know, herbs are primarily healers for the human body.

There are a variety of ways the cabbage can be eaten. Not only is the cabbage steamed, it is also an ingredient in many side dishes.

One of the green leafy foods that should always be included in menus, cabbage provides what is needed to help prevent heart ailments. Nothing is more important than the foods that are good for the viability of the heart.

Cabbage is also one of the few vegetables that can be cultivated in one's own garden. The wide rich looking leaves add beauty and color to the environment. Cabbage can be grown in three colors; green, purple and red.

16

Cantaloupe (melon)

Minerals: Calcium, Phosphorus
Vitamins: A

Very high in vitamin A, the fruit cantaloupe is also very effective in providing minerals for the body.

Cantaloupe is a melon. Melons come in a number of varieties, usually a sweet fruit. Melons offer a refreshing appeal to the human taste, especially since it is a natural fruit. Eaten fresh, the cantaloupe is very healthy.

Many people receive their needed minerals and vitamins through the taste of fresh natural food they like in particular. There is a wide variety of fresh fruits that are available to provide the normal healing vitamins the body needs.

The idea is, you should use natural foods such a fresh fruits as well as vegetables for the body to insure it receives what is needed in minerals and vitamins, through the taste you prefer in fruits and vegetables to maintain the health your body needs.

17

Carrots

Minerals: Potassium, Calcium, Phosphorus
Vitamins: A

Carrots are the most versatile of all the foods, in vitamins. It provides the body with a variety of minerals. Carrots do benefit the body in ways that can not be measured.

Carrots contain the minerals: calcium, copper, magnesium, potassium, sodium, sulfur, iron and chlorine.

Carrot juice also contains a variety of the vitamins the body will use regular, which includes the Vitamins A, B, C, D, E and G.

The carrot, a vegetable, offers the body more minerals and vitamins combined, than any other single natural food.

The carrot could easily be considered one of the most healthy foods for the human body. As a snack—hot or cold, and a table vegetable, the carrot is an invaluable source of healing aids.

18

Cashew Nuts

Minerals: Phosphorus
Vitamins: B-Complex

Cashews, known as nuts, are relatively hard on the stomach, because of their difficulty to digest. One of the most widely known of the cashews is the pistachio.   The cashew tree bears more than the edible nut we are often familiar with. Other natural foods from the cashew tree include edible fruits such as the pear shaped cashew apples.

The cashew provides the body with phosphorus an absolute necessity for the proper formation of teeth and normal bone structure.

The most important mineral phosphorus, gives the body the required activity for nerves, including the stimulating of brain activity. Foods that do contain phosphorus can not be overlooked for the important role they play in providing the body with an essential mineral.

19

Cauliflower

Minerals: Calcium, Phosphorus
Vitamins: A

The structure of the teeth are directly related to the amount of calcium the body absorbs. If it is necessary to find a specific need for calcium that is overlooked, muscle contraction depends on the calcium in the body.

Cauliflower is a good natural food source of essential vitamins and minerals. Cauliflower can be used in a variety of ways in preparation as a food. A seasonal plant, cauliflower can become a substitute for other sources of the body's vitamins and minerals.

Calcium will lower the body's risk of developing heart disease. Often overlooked, cancer of the colon can be contributed to low levels or no level of calcium maintained in the body on a daily and regular basis. The blood pressure, can be lowered by maintaining a high level of calcium in the body. A wide variety of sources to receive calcium for the body can be a life saver.

20

Celery

Minerals: Calcium, Iron, Phosphorus
Vitamins: A, B, C

Celery is often eaten raw. Celery seeds are ground into celery salt. Used in soups and salads, celery is also cooked in a variety of ways. Celery has a very pleasant flavor and is crisp, when eaten.

The superior vitamin content of celery makes it a very nourishing food. Celery is a herb, grown throughout the world. Celery contains a multiple of vitamins and minerals that are essential to the body.

As a B-Vitamin, celery also contain the vitamins to help prevent ulcers. Very few foods provide the vitamins that help prevent a common ailment, such as ulcers. Adequate nutrition, by including natural foods such as celery in menus, help prevent varying diseases.

21

Cereal

Minerals: Phosphorus, Calcium
Vitamins: A

Cereal is exceptionally good for the body. Most cereal are in some form of the three best popular types; cheerios, wheaties or corn flakes.

It is the pure grain that provides what the body needs when it comes to cereal. Cereal are made directly from the natural food—grain.

Grain food comes in a wide variety of types—that is, the names associated with the different styles and brands of grain food available are numerous to choose from.

When they are cereal and are in any form of oats, wheat, or corn, they are generally going to provide the body with the necessary vitamins and minerals needed for good health.

22

Cherries

Minerals: Calcium, Phosphorus
Vitamins: A

Cherries are one of the most edible fruits cultivated. Cherries are sweet and provide a pleasing taste while giving the body needed nutrition.

Cherries are also known to be sour and are grown in many regions throughout the world.

The acid that is provided from the fruit, do provide a very high content of Vitamin A and a needed protection against the development of infections. Cherries also provide the sodium content the body has a need for, generally found in natural foods.

There are a wide variety of uses of cherries that include, salads and many desserts. Cherries are also used to make jam. Juice is also made from cherries to help provide an added method for people to receive the nutrition they need.

23

Chicken (poultry)

Minerals: Iron, Calcium, Phosphorus
Vitamins: B-12, Niacin

Chicken provides the body with protein and iron. Protein can also be acquired through foods that are not meat. Meat contains such a high level of protein, and is often considered the best source.

Chicken can not be over looked, cooked properly, it provides Vitamins B-12 and Niacin—that is not common in many foods. Often found in many soups, chicken is used as a healing food in stages of recovery for the body.

When the body is injured and in need of nutrients through vitamins or minerals for recovery, it becomes imperative to acquire the body's needed nutrients, form a variety of sources. Chicken in soup is one of the healthy choices to receive healing vitamins and minerals for the body.

24

Chives

Minerals: Sulfur
Vitamins: C

Few foods provide sulfur for the body. High in Vitamin C , chives are one of the edible foods that can be grown indoors.

There are a variety of uses for chives. They are widely known as a flavoring for various soups. Chives are also used to add flavor to omelets. In many cheese dishes, chives add an additional flavor. The leaves of the chive plant are used to assist in flavoring a variety of food dishes.

In some countries, chives grow as wild plants. A green vegetable, grown indoors, you can observe the lavender flowers it bears.

As a herb, this natural food serves a specific purpose in helping complete the variety of natural foods eaten for nutrition and as a healing food for the body.

25

Clams

Minerals: Phosphorus, Calcium
Vitamins: A

Clams are very high in Vitamin A, they are very high in phosphorus and very high in calcium.

Calcium is a necessity for the heart, in its ability to transmit impulses through the nerves, which is a part of a process in electric conduction inside the human body. Calcium do other wonders for the body. Calcium help prevent the development of heart disease, while it also reduces the risk of cancer. The body's blood pressure can also be lowered from the calcium inside the body. Calcium will help prevent strokes.

The body must relax at times in order to sleep. It is the calcium inside the body that help promote relaxation. When there is a high calcium content in the body, the risk of heats disease has been lowered tremendously.

26

Coconut

Minerals: Phosphorus, Calcium
Vitamins: C

Coconut is a fruit. Inside is a sweet milky fluid. The inside white "meat" of the coconut is dried for production. Most tropical regions depend on the coconut as a primary source of food. The entire coconut tree has value. Just about every part of the coconut tree is used for something related to food products. The outer fiber and leaves of the coconut tree are used for commercial products, due to their toughness and strength.

The coconut is often eaten as a snack. Coconut is a delicacy in the tropics. The root of the coconut tree is also a chewable product that is used in some regions. The central part of the coconut tree also offers an edible stem that provides a food in tropical countries. There is a natural beverage that is obtained from the coconut for drinking.

27

Cod (fish)

Minerals: Phosphorus, Calcium, Iron
Vitamins: A, C, Niacin

Cod fish is one of the healthiest fish known. The cod-liver oil that is well known as an omega-3 fatty acid, is rarely found in other foods that are widely eaten. Fish-oil do wonders in healing the body. Helping prevent cancer, this oil will thin the blood and prevent clogged arteries. The intense swelling and known stiffness as well as the pain from rheumatoid arthritis is relieved through the use of cod-liver oil.

The cod fish has a variety of species that are commonly known fish, valuable to the health of the human body. The Pollock and the haddock are two of the important species that are apart of the commercial fish market.

Cod-liver oil, which is Vitamin D for the body, contribute to the healing of the skin, which often receive its enriching vitamins from the natural sun, for improved health and beauty of the skin.

28

Corn

Minerals: Phosphorus, Calcium
Vitamins: A, B-6

High in Vitamin A, corn is also a good source of the mineral phosphorus. Corn will help provide fiber the body needs.

Corn is the most widely grown and cultivated crop in America. With a variety of uses, corn is popular as a snack, commonly known as popcorn. Corn is ground into meal, known as corn meal. Corn is a popular vegetable, eaten sweet with a variety of dishes and n many menus. Even the popular corn-on-the-cob is a widely known dish.

Corn provides the Vitamin B-6 known as pyridoxine. Good for aiding in the formation of blood cells, this is also needed for nerves and the body's metabolism. When the body is missing Vitamin B-6, it can result in problems such as depression, clogged arteries and even problems with weight abnormality.

29

Cottage Cheese

Minerals: Calcium, Phosphorus
Vitamins: B

Cheese is a nutritious food for the body. A dairy product, it comes in a variety of types generally made from some of the different types of milk.

Cottage cheese is an excellent source of good healthy food for the bones. This is one of the foods that can help prevent many aging ailments, due to a lack of calcium for the body.

One of the key healers for the body is riboflavin. A Vitamin B, which is not often available in all common foods eaten daily, specific foods that do offer B-Vitamins, are exceptionally good in maintaining excellent health, which contribute to one of the most important functions, the nervous system. B-Vitamins such as riboflavin is essential for the effective operation of the metabolism of all foods that enter the body. The Vitamin B-2 (Riboflavin) found in cottage cheese, will help prevent many ailments to the body.

30

Cranberries

Minerals: Calcium, Phosphorus
Vitamins: A, C

Cranberries contain ascorbic acid, which is found in Vitamin C. Vitamin C is needed for the body's tissues and to help prevent wrinkles in the skin. Vitamin A is essential to healthy mucus membranes, to prevent allergies. Cranberries comes in the form of juice. An alternate source to receive ascorbic acid for the body, cranberries help give the needed protection and health aid the various ligaments and the arteries need.

Vitamin C, which is necessary for growth during childhood, is also needed during the adult life of the body. Essential in ways that are often overlooked, high amounts of ascorbic acid do not harm the body, it helps provide the needed protection against infections.

The important needs of the body for ascorbic acid from many fruits help deposit the minerals the body needs even in the bones. Deposits of Vitamin C builds healthy cells throughout the body.

31

Cucumbers

Minerals: Phosphorus, Calcium
Vitamins: C

Cucumbers are life savers. A natural herb, the fruit can be eaten as a snack. The cucumber is a timely fruit and must be harvested at the appropriate moment to prevent over development, and a wasted crop.

Cucumbers are widely eaten and widely known as a common seasonal fruit. As an alternate or primary source of an essential vitamin for the body, there are a variety of ways the cucumber can be eaten. It is also widely known that cucumbers are pickled. The taste of the pickled cucumber has become a traditional favorite of many people.

Cucumbers will provide protection for the body in numerous ways. It is well known how Vitamin C is a protector for the immune system, in helping reduce the risk of infections inside the body. Using a variety of foods to help protect the body from developing diseases is a good practice.

32

Dates

Minerals: Calcium, Phosphorus
Vitamins: A

Dates are a source of a healthy food for some regions of the world. The fruit provides a source of protein for the body. The minerals provided from dates include calcium and phosphorus.

It is the high natural sugar content of the dates that also makes them a source of nutrition that natural foods provide for the body.

The brains activity depends on the amount of phosphorus the body receives. When there are disorders in the human body's nervous system, it is often lacking in the content of phosphorus. Even a weakness in strength of the human body itself, can be contributed to shortages of phosphorus.

Establishing a dislike for particular foods, especially the natural foods, can be harmful to the body. Being unaware of the vital nutrients the body needs, and the sources in which those minerals and vitamins can be obtained, is harmful.

33

Eggplant

Minerals: Phosphorus, Calcium
Vitamins: A

The eggplant is a fruit. They are common in a variety of different shapes and colors. Eggplants are grown very similar to the tomato.

As a source of Vitamin A, eggplants offer an alternate source of the needed vitamin that help improve the skin, hair, nails and gums.

In fruits, Vitamin A contain beta-carotene, which will help prevent lung disease, due to the antioxidant contained in this fruit. Heart disease risk is lowered when the Vitamin A is obtained from beta-carotene.

Eggplants are generally lower in nutrients than other fruits, however, they do provide an alternate source of other vital minerals and vitamins to the body. Used often for many people that want a variety of foods, the eggplant is one of the few that can be considered vital as an alternate source of healthy foods the body is in absolute need of to help prevent diseases.

34

Fish

Fish-oil is the nutrition that is compatible to the omega-3 fatty acid that will help prevent cancer and heart disease.

Some of the most common fish found in the supermarket that are considered nutritious for the human body includes:

- Anchovies
- Bass
- Clams
- Cod
- Flounder
- Haddock
- Lobster
- Oysters
- Perch
- Pollack
- Salmon
- Sardines
- Trout
- Tuna
- White fish

This list represent some of the fish that are sources of cod-liver oil and fish oil, that can help heal the body.

35

Fruit

Nothing quite takes the place of fruit in what it can do to enhance the good health of the human body. What does fruit really do for the body? Most everyone is aware of the natural vitamins fruits provide for the body.

There is a wide variety of fruits. The many vitamins they provide, makes it impossible to list them all. In general, the fruits that are available in season and conveniently in your area can be a good choice.

Fruits restore to the body, the needed minerals and vitamins that provide the nutrients that are necessary for proper energy and health.

A variety of fruits are good for the body. Fruits add a boost and give the body it's energy, and comfort to the entire system of the body. The body can be kept in excellent health, when you provide a variety of natural foods containing nutrients that are essential for the body.

Most fruits do contain some form of natural acid. When eaten, fruits will help prevent infections and diseases from developing inside the body.

36

Grapes

Minerals: Calcium, Phosphorus
Vitamins: A, C

Grapes are one of the most widely edible fruits in the world. Grapes as a natural food go back to the beginning of time. Grapes are healthy for the body. A variety of food products are produced from the grape. As an option, grape comes in juice , jelly and canned.

Grapes can help prolong your life. The acid inside the grape heals the body while providing a protective mechanism to help prevent diseases.

As a snack many grapes are sweet and soothing in taste. Many seedless grapes are eaten in their raw state.

Grapes come in many different sizes, colors, and shapes—all of them perform the same function, especially for providing the body with the needed natural minerals and vitamins that can heal the body very effectively.

37

Garlic

Minerals: Selenium
Vitamins: B-Complex (Biotin)

Garlic is a very strong herb. A healer for the body in a variety of ways, garlic is a known medicine for the digestive system. Garlic has also been known to help prevent heart disease.

Garlic has a very strong odor and a very strong taste. The high potency of garlic an antioxidant helps prevent cancer.

Garlic is actually a fruit. The small seeds that make it a fruit, have been cultivated as far back as time is known. Garlic is definitely a natural medicine for the human body—it is better known for flavoring in cooking, and as a digestive stimulant.

The mineral selenium helps protect the heart and the immune system of the body. Selenium helps protect the body against cancer that can occur in the lungs and the colon. The body's aging process slows with selenium.

38

Grapefruit

Minerals: Sodium, Potassium
Vitamins: C

Grapefruit is an absolute good food. Providing a very high potassium content, the heart is dramatically improved in health by regular consumption of grapefruit.

How does grapefruit heal the body? Grapefruit is high in acidity. The natural content of acid from the fruit help destroy any bacteria that builds inside the body. It is bacteria that ultimately develop diseases inside the body. Grapefruit also comes in the form of juice that can be purchased in single servings as well as large reusable sizes. The grapefruit is invaluable to the human body. A large pink in color hull, the grapefruit, when fresh can offer a sweet taste as a very pleasing fruit. One of the most edible fruits throughout the world, as a natural food, the grapefruit is a traditional natural fruit that is excellent in healing the body and it provides protection against many common infections.

39

Greens

Minerals: Calcium, Phosphorus, Iron
Vitamins: A, C

Collard greens—Mustard greens—Turnip greens

These are the most common greens that are eaten as natural foods. Greens are healthy for the human body. Turnips are high in calcium and can help prevent cancer. The greens can be eaten or the turnip. The turnip resemble a small potato, and is very high in sodium.

The mustard green, a dark green leaf, is an herb. Herbs do provide a natural medicine that can heal the human body. The mustard green comes in a variety of plants. Most common are the table mustard, leafy, an edible green that will provide needed nutrition. Very high in Vitamin A, greens are an excellent source of nutrition for the body.

Turnip greens are another widely edible vegetable. Often cooked and seasoned to taste, this herb will do wonders in giving the body the healing medicine it needs, as do many dark green leafy vegetables.

40

Haddock (fish)

Minerals: Phosphorus, Calcium
Vitamins: B-12

Fish is considered an excellent food. The Vitamin B-12 is one of the critical vitamins, the human body needs. When there is no natural food that is eaten regularly to acquire this important vitamin, eating haddock can provide this needed and essential vitamin. Vitamin B-12 is good for the nervous system. How you feel, has a lot to do with the body's intake and supply of the Vitamin B-12 (cobalamin) needed for all living cells.

Some natural foods do provide the essential nutrients the body needs. When you are unaware of the foods that do provide the essential needs of the body and do not receive them, then ailments set in. People are often sick and totally unaware of the condition their body is in. Most of the time the body is lacking in minerals, vitamins and nutrients that are absolutely essential to maintain good health.

41

Herbs

What are herbs? Herbs are plants that provide some type of medical property as its source. Pronounced with the "h" silent, herbs are healers for the human body. Why are herbs mentioned here? Simply because herbs are found in many natural foods we eat.

When it is mentioned that there is some type of healing property found in food, as you may know—medicine is that part of science that deals with the practice of healing the body. When herbs are used, they coincide with the medical principles of healing.

Herbs can do wonders for the body. Knowing which herbs to aid particular and specific ailments is actually beyond the scope of this book. However, many herbs in the natural foods, are mentioned in this study.

Always remember, it is the natural foods themselves that provide the healing mechanism the body need in nutrients, minerals and vitamins that restore the body to its original energy level and proper health.

42

Honey

Minerals: Phosphorus
Vitamins: B-3 (Niacin)

Honey does something for the body to help relieve pain. Sweet naturally, there are a variety of uses of honey as an ingredient in cooking.

As a sweetener, honey can be used in many natural drinks to add taste. The enzymes and oils that are found in honey provides an essential mineral the body can use. Niacin, aids the digestive system, improves blood circulation and help prevent heart disease.

Honey is a natural sweet and thick saturated sugar solution taken from the nectar of flowers. Honey is also extracted from buckwheat. The many varieties of honey are generally based on the age of the honey. The time that is allowed for the honey to age is directly related to the color of the honey, as well as the flavor.

Honey should not be overlooked for its content of phosphorus, when other natural foods are not appealing.

43

Honeydew (melon)

Minerals: Calcium, Phosphorus
Vitamins: A, C

People love honeydew. A seasonal melon, it is sweet and provide a good source of natural Vitamin A, and Vitamin C. Melons come in a variety of types, the honeydew is just one of the many widely eaten melons.

Commonly known to many honeydew can help prevent eating manufactured sweets. Too often, processed sweets can contain too much refined sugar that can be harmful to the human body, especially as the body ages, and many organs wear out, then become weak in their processing of sugar products. The honeydew can become a seasonal fruit when other summer melons are out of season.

Melons are a high water content fruit. As a perishable food, the honeydew is a better preserved fruit due to the harder rinds, than many other melons.

44

Juice

Mixed juices and vegetable juices are the key to absolute good health. There are a variety of juices that are good for the body. When good natural foods can not be eaten, juice is the next best thing to acquire a healthy source of minerals and vitamins. Three of the best known juices for the body's health are grape juice, orange juice and cranberry juice. Natural foods contain juice that do provide exactly what the body needs.

Juices can be made from raw vegetables too. Using a juicer, a combination of many common juices can cure ailments that are the direct result of the body's lack of specific nutrients, minerals or vitamins. When purchased, most juicers do provide a list and combination of fruits as well as vegetables that can be used to make a variety of juices that are an absolute necessity for the body.

Other extremely healthy juices to keep in mind include: tomato juice and grapefruit juice.

45

Ketchup

Ketchup is a combination of tomatoes and vinegar. Both of the two are exceptionally good for the body in providing the healing nutrients the body needs. The vinegar in ketchup makes this and ideal healer. Ketchup, directly from the tomato, offers Vitamins A and C to the body. Used for a variety of cooking and tasty dishes, this is one of the most healthy foods to include. As a spread-on, a dip and a cooking item, few foods contain the dual nutritious value and high protection that ketchup gives the body.

Ketchup can help prevent heart disease. Ketchup contains two foods, tomatoes and vinegar that are unmatched in a combination of natural foods.

The tomato provides the type of acid that a natural food can give to keep diseases from developing in the body. When a second acid is even added to tomatoes, through the use of vinegar, they produce a one named food that is hard to match in protection to a vital organ, the heart.

46

Kiwifruit

Minerals: Potassium
Vitamins: C

Kiwi as a fruit is also known as gooseberry kiwifruit, which helps prevent esophageal cancer. Kiwi is the fruit to buy. This fruit can help prevent high blood pressure. A small edible fruit with a colorful green distinctive flesh, the kiwi is sweet and tasty. Kiwi can be eaten raw as a natural fruit or it can be cooked. Few fruits can improve the overall internal refreshing of the body than the kiwi. Kiwi is a refreshing fruit, that allows the internal seeds that surround the inner core of the fruit to be eaten.

The potassium in Kiwi will help lower the body's blood pressure. When the body needs potassium, it leads to heart problems. The nerves and muscles in the body depend on a regular supply of potassium.

47

Lamb

Minerals: Calcium, Phosphorus, Iron
Vitamins: A

Lamb quarters are extremely high in Vitamin A. Lamb is not considered one of the natural foods, it is a meat.

Meat offers the body protein. Very high in protein, lamb provides an abundance of a needed vitamin. The primary reason many meats do provide the high protein they offer, is due to the food animals eat.

Animals are generally raised on grain food. Grain food as we know is good in a variety of natural foods for the human body. As the grain foods are eaten, by animals, it gives their skin nutrients. When the meat of is eaten, the body receives protein the animal has obtained to grow their bodies.

48

Lemons

Minerals: Calcium, Phosphorus, Potassium
Vitamins: C
Vitamin C destroy infections inside the body. Lemons do provide the Vitamin C needed to stay healthy. Here is a list of the many ailments, high contents of Vitamin C will help prevent:

·   Allergies
·   Arthritis
·   Cancer
·   Heart disease
·   Liver disease
·   Lung disease
·   Skin disease
·   Ulcers
·   Tooth decay
·   Gland infections

Lemons provide ascorbic acid that can help to prevent bacteria that accumulate inside the body to form diseases.

The lemon is a fruit. An outer color that is a pale-yellow, lemons contain a vitamin, citrin. Lemon, a citrus fruit is also used as a flavoring in cooking.

49

Lettuce

Minerals: Sodium, Calcium, Phosphorus
Vitamins: A

Lettuce is another natural food good for the body. One of the most widely cultivated plants, lettuce comes in many varieties. The most common the head lettuce, is a very healthy natural food, providing the body with needed sodium, calcium and phosphorus.

The most common types of lettuce are the head lettuce, leaf lettuce, romaine lettuce and the asparagus lettuce.

Lettuce is highly commercialized. Just about every restaurant use lettuce in some form. Lettuce can also be grown in the home garden.

The wide use of lettuce makes it so popular as a natural food, it may be the only natural food that is grown widely, repeatedly and in abundance.

As a herb, the lettuce can be eaten raw, to give the body essential nutrients. Calcium, found in lettuce, is known to lower the body's risk of developing heart disease.

50

Limes

Minerals: Calcium, Potassium
Vitamins: A, C

Limes contain an acid that will protect the body against diseases. As a fruit, limes are extremely healthy as a nutritious food.

Prior to the invention of vitamins, lime was used to prevent and cure the disease, scurvy.

Limes are mostly grown and cultivated for the juice. Similar to lemons in size, a green oval to spherical shape, the fruit grows on trees in most tropical regions.

Limes can be included as an exceptional fruit, to help provide the body with preventive medicine that is natural, in giving the body needed acid to fight any potential bacteria infection.

51

Lobster

Minerals: Phosphorus, Calcium
Vitamins: A, B-3 (Niacin), B-12 (Cobalamin)

What does lobster provide that the body needs? Lobster is a seafood with the needed vitamin cobalamin. Vitamin B-12, cobolamin, contributes to the body's nervous system—which is a necessary vitamin, essential for every living cell in the body.

Niacin and B-12 can not be found in many foods. It is absolutely imperative to locate foods that can provide a mineral or vitamin that is not plentiful in other foods, to provide needed nutrition for the body.

Although, calcium phosphorus and Vitamin A are necessary, they are also common in plenty of the other variety of foods.

Once a food is found to be healthy for the body, and it provides something that is an absolute necessity for the body's health, a serious interest should be taken in that food.

52

Mangoes

Minerals: Sodium
Vitamins: A, C

Mango is a fruit that provides good nutrition for the body. The evergreen tree grows in tropical regions throughout the world.

The egg shaped mango is a soft juicy fruit that has a spicy taste. Mangoes can be eaten as a dessert or added to fruit salads.

Mango is very high in Vitamin A, providing the beta-carotene, one of the antioxidants that is beneficial to the body in numerous ways, protecting the body against infections by providing the body with a very high resistance. When the body lacks the needed amount of Vitamin A, the results can often be reflected in poor vision.

The sodium that is provided through mango, is needed because the body looses its sodium content from the bladder and during perspiration.

53

Milk

Minerals: Calcium, Phosphorus, Iron, Protein, Magnesium, Iodine
Vitamins: A, C, D

Milk is widely known to provide the necessary calcium the body needs for good bone structure and nourishment.

Milk is extremely high in calcium. There are other essential minerals and vitamins for the body found in milk, such as; biotin, folic acid, riboflavin and Vitamin B-12, all known for healing the body, while preventing a variety of aliments.

Milk is also very high in casein. When milk can be consumed in abundance, it provides too much casein and can cause excessive mucus, runny noses and even congestion in the chest when consumption is too high.

Other good sources of milk are: soybean, sesame seeds, almonds and pecans. Goat milk is an option for those with sensitive digestive systems.

54

Mushrooms

Minerals: Phosphorus, Calcium
Vitamins: B-12, Niacin

What can mushrooms do to help heal the body? Mushrooms do provide a very high amount of phosphorus. Phosphorus is important and can be extremely high in specific foods, and it can be overlooked for it's importance to the human body.

High in Vitamin B-12 and niacin, mushrooms offer amino acid to the body, which will help prevent diseases such as cancer.

Mushrooms are cooked in a variety of ways and can be included in a variety of menus. Mushrooms do come in a wide choice of species even through they are all bitter and tasteless, with one specific nutlike flavor, they are all cultivated separately.

Not all mushrooms are edible. Those that are cultivated and processed for eating can be very fresh when they are grown for commercial use. Canning of mushrooms is widely practiced throughout the world.

55

Oatmeal

Minerals: Phosphorus, Calcium
Vitamins: B-1 (Thiamine)

Oatmeal provides fiber to the body. Oats are known to help lower the body's cholesterol level.

Oats are a grain food. There are many varieties of commonly known grains or seeds that comprise the many oats that are edible.

There are many uses of oats too, in addition to the wide range of food choices that we have to include for oats.

Oatmeal is generally eaten as a hot, prepared dish. Many people eat oatmeal as a breakfast dish. Oats are especially high in protein. People often look for sources of protein when they limit their intake of meat. Oatmeal provides nutrition that includes a source of thiamin, generally known as Vitamin B-1. Thiamine is a B-Vitamin that is a benefit to the body's mental and brain activity. Thiamine enhances the body's energy level too.

56

Okra

Minerals: Phosphorus, Calcium
Vitamins: A

Okra is a green vegetable that is often used in soups and stews. Eaten separately, okra will provide an alternate source of Vitamin A. The body needs phosphorus to maintain a healthy bone structure for your entire life. Calcium also provides the needed minerals to help keep the teeth healthy. Calcium will help the body to relax and sleep with adequate rest. When calcium is kept high inside the body, it can also lower the risk of heart disease.

Using more that one source to receive the nutrients essential for the body can help break the monotony of other foods. Knowing nutritious foods can help to insure the daily intake of food is healthy.

Vitamin A should never be underestimated for its importance to good health. The beta-carotene in foods is what helps the body produce Vitamin A to keep the body's resistance high to fight infections.

57

Olives

Minerals: Calcium, Phosphorus
Vitamins: A

The olive tree bears a small fruit that many people eat as a snack. The unique taste of the olive offer another source of Vitamin A for the body.

Vitamin A should not be overlooked, because it provides an antioxidant that protects the body against infections. Vitamin A will help prevent the development of lung disease. Olives not only provide us with a fruit, it also provides a very healthy oil. Olive oil, which is taken from the olive, is widely used in cooking.

The green olive that is unripe when harvested, is often preserved in oil as an edible fruit. When olives are fully ripe, they become a dark blush color. After picking those dark blue olives, they turn blackish and retain that color through canning.

58

Onions

Minerals: Calcium, Phosphorus
Vitamins: A

The onion is an herb. Herbs are known as natural medicine to heal the human body. Onions help prevent heart disease. The onion may be one of the most versatile vegetables in the world.

Many people eat onions raw, in salads and often as slices, similar to other vegetables while consuming a meal.

Onions are used in many ways commonly known, in soups, stews, and as flavor or seasoning in cooking.

Rarely are people aware of the high value onions offer in the acid it contains in helping prevent the accumulation of bacteria, which contribute to the development of diseases.

Onions are a year round crop. They can be obtained fresh at almost anytime. Onions come in a wide variety and they are all good in helping heal the body.

59

Oranges

Minerals: Calcium, Phosphorus
Vitamins: A, C

The orange is known to be a good source of Vitamin C, and they are also a very good source of Vitamin A.

These two vitamins found in oranges and orange juice, help cure allergies. Keeping the gland cells healthy is done by rich amounts of Vitamins A and C.

Many people are unaware that their ailments in many cases are due directly to the body's lack of minerals and vitamins that fight-off the bacteria that harm the human body.

Foods that are high in vitamins like the orange, help prevent a variety of common ailments that are taken for granted. These vitamins improve the eyesight, improve the skin, help prevent ulcers, keep the teeth healthy and provide the needed protection for the heart and liver.

60

Parsley

Minerals: Phosphorus, Calcium
Vitamins: A

Parsley contain one of the highest amounts of Vitamin A in a natural food. Vitamin A will heal a variety of ailments, and promotes healthy skin, hair, bone growth, finger nails and help prevent cancer.

Parsley is a flower like plant. Generally used as flavoring and a seasoning in many food recipes, parsley comes in a variety of species.

Along with its variety of uses, parsley can be found on a different number of crops. A uniform looking flower, the parsley leaf is found on common known vegetables such as carrots and celery, two of the important natural foods for the body.

Parsley is an herb that is often used medically to help in healing the body. Vitamins needed to strengthen the internal system of the human body can come directly from parsley.

61

Pasta

Minerals: Manganese, Iron, Phosphorus, Calcium, Zinc
Vitamins: A

Is pasta healthy for your body? Pasta is a healthy food that is low in fat and provides the body with a variety of nutritious minerals.

Pasta comes in a variety of types, generally known most commonly in the making of spaghetti. The zinc and magnesium that is in the pasta are two of the body's important minerals. Magnesium will lower blood pressure and can reduce the risk of strokes. Zinc, which is also a mineral from pasta, can help prevent cancer.

Pasta is not all carbohydrates. In addition to carbohydrates are other very important minerals that are not found in many other foods. Eaten in moderation pasta can help heal and dramatically improve your health as a nutritious food for the body.

62

Peaches

Minerals: Phosphorus, Calcium, Potassium
Vitamins: A, C

Potassium is a necessity to the body for good health. The proper function of the nerves in the body require the use of potassium, which is found in peaches.

Peaches are a great snack while they add the body with needed nutrients that heal the entire body. Peaches offer sodium to the body, a salt necessary for life to exist. Peaches are canned, made into jam, preserves, and often frozen too.

Eaten in moderation, peaches also provide the cells and membrane with the needed potassium, which help them functioning at their optimum levels for good overall health and protection.

The nerves, muscles and the body's balance of fluids depend on the intake of potassium that also help the body's acid balance for proper health. Peaches can also be a good substitute for other fruits, to help provide Vitamin C, especially during the period of colds and influenza.

63

Peas

Minerals: Phosphorus, Calcium
Vitamins: A, C

Peas come in a variety of types. The green pea provides a high degree of vitamins. Peas are also known by field peas—while both are natural foods. Sources of minerals and vitamins for the body, peas are where the body receives it source of enzymes. These vegetables are extremely good for the body when first cooked and hot. As the heat is retained while vegetables sit, they loose their full value of total vitamins. Therefore, it is imperative to eat vegetables that are cooked immediately, while they are steam hot.

Canned peas are also a good substitute for the fresh cooked raw peas. Even though the canned peas contain less vitamins than the fresh peas, the sources of what the body use are still contained in canned peas, only in a smaller quantity of vitamins.

64

Pears

Minerals: Phosphorus, Calcium, Iodine
Vitamins: A, C, B-Complex

Pear trees bear a natural fruit that is juicy. Pears are in many different varieties. The region in which pears are grown will help determine their distinctive taste.

Pears provide the body with needed iodine. Iodine helps control the body's metabolism. It assist in burning excess fat from the body.

B-Complex provides the body with the necessary carbohydrates that are essential in the body through the metabolism process. B-Complex as a vitamin can often be overlooked. B-Complex is important for proper cell growth, the body's reproduction system and the prevention of heart attacks.

As a fruit containing a triple source of vitamins, the value to the body is beneficial in numerous ways through the healing of wounds and damaged tissues while helping rebuild the body and restore deficiencies, that are critical to good health.

65

Pecan

Minerals: Phosphorus, Calcium, Iron
Vitamins: A

Pecans are an edible fruit that most people are totally familiar with. Iron in pecans provide what every cell in the body depends on to receive a normal supply of oxygen to maintain life.

One of the most commercialized fruits there is, pecans have uses that are almost unimaginable in cooking and recipes.

Because the pecan is so widely known, a great deal can be said on its nutritious value. There are varieties of pecans throughout the world. Used as a snack and in every possible method that can add a taste unique to the pecan, there is no limit to the continued use of the pecan as a source of healthy natural food.

It is the natural fruits that help restore the body's needed nutrients for the purpose of maintaining excellent health. The pecan is one of the natural sources of human healing foods.

66

Peppers (green)

Minerals: Calcium, Phosphorus
Vitamins: A

Green peppers come in a variety of types as a natural food. The bell pepper is very high in Vitamin A. Peppers do provide a needed natural nutrition to the body.

It is commonly known that green peppers do provide the body with the necessary minerals that stimulate the fossils in the growth of the hair by helping the oil to remain in the scalp that promotes growth.

Green peppers have a variety of uses, it is difficult to avoid peppers as an inclusion in some type of menu.

The green pepper plant is also used to develop one of the world's leading spices, pepper. Green peppers as a whole are also used as spice seasoning and flavor in many dishes through cooking.

Green peppers are also herbaceous plants.

67

Peppers (red)

The red pepper is actually the same type of herb as the black pepper. Pepper is one of the worlds oldest spices. The red pepper is the black pepper, with its outer covering removed.

The table use of pepper should be as a seasoning and not as a spicy covering for taste. The abundance of black pepper to the human body can be harmful. Used in moderation, pepper can serve a meaningful purpose in the natural foods that are common in everyday cooking.

The pepper plant is grown throughout the world, and have some uses medically. There are specific ailments that can be cured by uses of the pepper plant.

As a naturally grown plant, peppers come in a variety of species.

Some areas of the world can grow more of the plants than others, due to moisture that aids the growth of pepper plants.

68

Perch (fish)

Minerals: Phosphorus, Calcium, Iron, Iodine, Magnesium
Vitamins: B-1, B-2, B-3, E

The perch is another fish that will provide good nutrition for the body. The perch is found in many shallow lakes and ponds.

The fish oil can be a very good source for the body to reduce pain from ailments such as arthritis and even inflammation.

The body's joints need the fatty acids that are present in various mineral oils that will heal the body. The cod-liver oil that is found in fish, provides omega-e fatty acid that will strengthen many of the body's cells against the bacteria that leads to cancer.

The fish oil can also help prevent arteries from clogging, something that can often lead to heart failure.

Diseases that develop inside the body are primarily due to the body's lack of the agents in minerals and vitamins that destroy unwanted bacteria. Eating fish will provide oils that will help prevent the development of cancer.

69

Pineapples

Minerals: Manganese
Vitamins: A, C

Pineapple comes fresh, canned and in juice. The manganese our body needs will keep the body resistance high. Many illnesses are due to low body resistance to fight-off infection and germs.

The pineapple is a unique natural food. Grown in the tropics, the fruit offers fiber for the body. As a domesticated plant, the pineapple is a sweet juicy fruit. The pineapple grows from its water-holding tank located at the very bottom of the plant, similar to that of a tank reservoir. Nothing quite matches the natural growth of the pineapple. The covered leaves act as a catch-basin for the bottom tanks of water that provides the source of growth for the plant.

Manganese for the human body, keeps the metabolism and muscle coordination very active.

70

Plums

Minerals: Phosphorus, Calcium
Vitamins: A (Beta-Carotene)

Plums are a natural fruit that is sweet and rich in the supply of sugar for the body. Natural sugar for the body is a necessity. Vitamin A that is also found in the plum offers the body the antioxidant needed to help prevent infections.

Beta-carotene found in this fruit coverts to Vitamin A inside the body, then protect the body from the development of cancer. Vitamins can help do wonders for the body especially when they come from natural foods.

Vitamin A is stored inside the liver of the body, then released as it is needed to help protect the body. Vitamin A contributes to good eyesight. A deficiency of Vitamin A gives off signs of such ailments as dry skin, or allergies. Even fatigue of the body can be contributed to a lack of Vitamin A inside the body.

A high resistance to infections can be contributed to high amounts of Vitamin A stored inside the body.

71

Pollack (fish)

Minerals: Calcium, Phosphorus, Iodine
Vitamins: A, C

Fish offers the body oil that will help fight diseases and prevent infections. Body tissues are repaired when the body absorbs the fighting agents such as cod-liver oil and fish oil.

The minerals iron and iodine found in fish also help protect the immune system of the body. Pollack contains the omega-3 fatty acid the body uses to fight cancer in the body.

The iodine found in fish, is stored inside the human body to assist the body's metabolism. This iodine can help in the destruction of excess fat through the digestive process. The use of iodine by the body will improve the reproductive system, promote the growth of hair and even improve the skin. The body's growth and continued health is dependent on the mineral, iodine.

72

Pomegranates

Minerals: Phosphorus
Vitamins: Biotin

The pomegranate seed offer healing aids to the human body. A fruit, the pomegranate is a small tree that grows a fruit that is red in color and the size of an orange. Pomegranates are medically used for the treatment of tapeworm infections.

Biotin is a B-Complex vitamin that helps convert amino acid in the body from protein to the needed sugar for the body.

Inside the pomegranate is a sweet edible pulp that contain an acid, nutritious for the human body. A tree or shrub, the pomegranate is as old as time and goes back to the origin of cultivation with ancient times.

With its beautiful red flowers and glossy leaves, the pomegranate is a cultivated fruit throughout the world.

73

Potatoes (Irish)

Minerals: Phosphorus, Calcium
Vitamins: A, C

The Irish potato is a starch. It is also an herb. Grown from the ground this natural food can provide needed nutrients for the human body when properly prepared.

As a fruit, the potato is cultivated throughout the world. Many states are generally well known for their high production of the Irish potato.

The potato can be eaten the year round. Cultivation of the Irish potato vary from different locations.

The Irish potato do provide valuable natural nutrients for the body. The Irish potato is high in water content, starch, carbohydrates and a very small percent of fat. Starch is used repeatedly by the body. Carbon and hydrogen will help build the body's energy.

74

Poultry

Poultry is a meat that is most common to us from fish, chicken and turkey. Fish is absolutely good for the body in providing minerals. Potassium is found in a variety of fish. Fish is good for keeping blood cholesterol and blood pressure at a low level in the body.

Fish is high in protein—it also provides iron and zinc for the body. A low calorie food when cooked properly poultry contain sodium and niacin.

Another high mineral found in fish is potassium. The lack of potassium in the body leads to sleeplessness and diminish your ability to remain alert. Vitamin D is also found in fish. When the body contain this vitamin, it helps the intake of calcium and phosphorus to the body.

Also found in poultry is magnesium, another mineral that is essential for the body. Magnesium is needed to help relax the body's nerves. Magnesium can help lower blood pressure and reduce the chances of a heart attack as well as help prevent clogged arteries.

75

Prunes

Minerals: Phosphorus, Calcium
Vitamin: A

Prunes offer fiber to the body. When fiber enters the body, it helps prevent bacteria from surviving inside the body. Eliminating bacteria, will help prevent the development of diseases.

Prunes can be eaten as a snack. They are often included in fruit salads. Prunes can be included in other menus.

Prunes are considered an ancient fruit. Cultivated years before many other popular fruits became common, the prune has been eaten for decades. Prunes come in the common purplish—blue color that is most widely known. There are other varieties of plumes, with the original colors, yellow, red and green. Plum trees are actually the species that originate the prune. The prune is a very healthy fruit for the human body. Prune juice is also an optional method to receive the minerals and vitamins from the fruit.

76

Pumpkins

Minerals: Phosphorus
Vitamins: A

The pumpkin is a very healthy natural fruit. A seasonal fruit, the pumpkin is very similar to the squash. Grown and cultivated widely throughout the world, the pumpkin can offer the body a very good source of needed natural Vitamin A, known to help keep the body's resistance to infections very high. Vitamin A generally contribute to healthy gums, skin and hair for the body. The eyesight is improved with the inclusion of this vitamin, which often comes in the form of beta-carotene, an antioxidant.

Antioxidants help reduce the risk of cancer and a preventive measure to strokes. Improving the arteries, beta-carotene help prevent heart attacks.

The pumpkin is also very high in fiber. Some foods are an exceptional source of nutrients that are a good protection for the body—pumpkin is one of those foods.

77

Radishes

Minerals: Calcium, Phosphorus
Vitamins: A, C

Radishes are generally eaten raw. An excellent natural food for the body, it is the root of the radish that makes it an edible food.

There are a variety of radishes in size and color. From small to large in a variety of shapes and colored in white, red or yellow, the radish is a herb for the body. Foods that are natural as a herb do provide the body with an agent that will quickly treat ailments by supplying needed nutrients.

A garden product, radish can be grown at home. They can be used in a variety of cooking recipes, including boiled for their softness, to chew.

Never overlook the importance the radish play as a health food to help keep the body replenished in minerals and vitamins.

78

Raisins

Minerals: Phosphorus, Calcium
Vitamins: A

Raisins provide a protection for the body that help prevent infections and the development of heart disease. Raisins are used in baking as well as a tasty fruit in warm cereal, such as oatmeal.

Raisins do for the body what many other foods can not do. A high source of the bet-carotene, which provide the body with Vitamin A, this is another one of those antioxidants that help protect the body against cancer.

It is the beta-carotene that help the internal body from developing lung cancer. Fighting the development of bacteria that leads to infections is a serious measure and precaution for good health—raisins can give the body this needed protection.

79

Rice

Minerals: Magnesium, Phosphorus, Iron, Iodine
Vitamins: B-Complex, E, K

Rice offers a different vitamin for the body. As a herb, rice is another one of the oldest cultivated crops in the world.

A nutritious grain food that comes in many varieties, it is the brown rice that provides the best nutrition for the body.

Too much white rice can cause a deficiency in the body. The brown rice contain bran, which is a vitamin rich portion covering the rice. When rice is white in color, the bran has been bleached away. Often you can hear the comment, brown rice is better for you.

Why rice is good for the human body is in the many minerals as well as the special vitamins the body receive. Rice is a natural food that grows in abundance. Rice is most commonly grown in climates where the temperature is warm and the climate is moist.

80

Salmon (fish)

Minerals: Phosphorus, Calcium
Vitamins: A, B-12 (Cobalamin)

Salmon is known for its concentration of B-12, a vitamin that is not found in many foods, however, it is needed for all the body's cells.

As a fresh water fish, salmon is a widely eaten poultry. Less harmful to the digestive system that heavier meats, fish can offer the body some added nutrition.

The salmon is a special family of fish, known for its orange-red color of its flesh. A migratory fish, that alters between fresh and salt water, the true salmon are often located in lakes as well as the sea.

There are a variety of species of salmon and they all offer the high degree of vitamins common to the King Salmon, one of the most popular species.

Salmon is also a canned fish. Salmon will offer the body a healthy dose of the vitamin known to help improve the nervous system.

81

Sardines

Minerals: Iodine, Phosphorus, Calcium
Vitamin: A

Sardines are a canned fish. Widely known for canning in factories, the sardine is a true healer for the human body. The iodine that this fish gives the body, makes it a healthy and nourishing food.

Helping prevent heart disease, lowering blood level and blood cholesterol level, few foods can provide the type of protection for the body as the sardine. The sardine is one of the most widely eaten foods in North America. These small fish, are easy to obtain, they reside through swimming at the very top near the surface of the water. Found both in fresh water and saltwater, the sardine can be a heavily salted fish in taste.

The fatty acids that are provided to the body from fish oil, do help heal the body by reducing pain from arthritis and inflammation.

82

Soups

One of the most important things a person can do for their body is include soup in their menus. What is soup? Soup is a combination of foods that are known healing foods. Combined for taste and many herbs added for distinct flavor, soup can be one of the most nutritious foods for the body.

Vegetable soup is one of the most widely eaten soups. The body receives a variety of natural minerals and vitamins through soup. Soup should be included, in meals as often as possible, even as a side dish.

Many times, people only consume soup when there is definitely an ailment that exist in the body. If eaten as a normal way of life and included in the course of the meal, soup can become a permanent source of receiving added minerals and vitamins that can protect the body.

Soup comes in a variety of types. Soup can be purchased to suit your taste. Common name soups found in the supermarket all include a variety of vegetables, and most are prepared with the best healing foods in mind.

83

Soybeans

Minerals: Calcium, Phosphorus, Iron
Vitamins: A, B-2 (Riboflavin)

Soybeans are herbs, a natural food that is high in protein and highly nutritious. Soybeans come as green vegetables or a dried bean that is often boiled or baked and for soup making.

Soybean is one of the most widely cultivated foods in the world. Vitamin B, makes soybean a very nutritious food for the body.

The riboflavin in soybean, a B-2 Vitamin, helps promote proper cell formation in the body, as well as healthy skin and hair. Iron will improve red blood cells improving the oxygen carrying capacity in the body. Minerals are an essential part of the healing process of the body. When the fiber that is contained in soybean enters the body, it will lower the blood cholesterol level. Soybean plays a greater role in providing good health and needed healing vitamins for the human body.

84

Spinach

Minerals: Calcium, Phosphorus, Iron
Vitamins: A, B-2

Spinach contains iron for the body. The body needs iron on a daily basis. Iron for the body is generally provided through the meat that is eaten. The natural foods we eat also can provide the body with the needed iron that help restore health and keep the needed supply of iron that will heal the body.

When the body experience a shortage of the nutrients through minerals, or vitamins that it needs for normal health, many ailments, infections and even unhealthy bacteria develop in the body. The many diseases experienced in the body are due to a lack of the necessary nutrients that fight the development of bacteria in the body.

Spinach offer more than iron for the body, it is also a good source of Vitamin A and riboflavin. Foods that can provide a multiple of nutrients are exceptionally good for the body, when eaten regular.

85

Sprouts

Minerals: Phosphorus, Calcium
Vitamins: A, C

Sprouts can be easily considered on of the most important foods the is. Healthy in a variety of ways, and especially a healing food for the body sprouts are commonly known by beans, an easily reproductive food.

Sprouts that are green beans and soybeans provide added nutrition that is uncommon in the healing process of the human body. Vitamins that are most effective in sprouts are Vitamins A and C.

Sprouts come from the growing of natural foods that are widely known to us as beans, oats and are often dried. Grain food is often referred to as wheat or rye in many of the foods we eat today. These seeded products are the foundation to the sprouted foods that are extremely healthy for the body in providing a high degree of nutrition.

Sprouts are used in many combination of food dishes that include a variety of vegetables and other recipes that should not be overlooked.

86

Squash

Minerals: Iron, Phosphorus, Calcium
Vitamins: A, C

Squash is an extremely healthy food that provides the body with good nutrition. Squash comes in a variety of types and may be seasonal, which limits purchases to specific times of the year.

What does squash do for the body? Squash as a fruit, offers the body the natural minerals and vitamins as agents that can give the body an additional source of iron.

Squash gives iron to the body that is needed for good mental health. Iron for the body provides the body cells with oxygen. The life of the body depends on iron.

Squash is produced the year round. There is a summer and winter squash which is not common in many fruits.

87

Strawberries

Minerals: Calcium
Vitamins: A

Strawberries as an herb, is one of the most edible fruits cultivated. A fruit that do provide calcium to the body, will help prevent lung cancer.

The calcium and Vitamin A in strawberries provide the body with the natural nutrients that help lower your risk of heart disease. Calcium help slow bone loss as the body ages. The antioxidant from Vitamin A is also a good protector for the body in preventing fatigue or even dry skin.

Strawberries are seasonal plants even though they are found the year round, due to the planting seasons varying in different regions.

Even though they are common the year round, the planting seasons vary in different regions.

Adding strawberries to a regular menu or as a snack can greatly improve body mechanisms such as the eyes, nerves, muscles, hair growth gums and your overall health.

88

Tangerines

Minerals: Calcium, Phosphorus
Vitamins: A, C

Tangerines are very high in Vitamin A. It is a high concentration of Vitamins A and C that help maintain healthy gland cells for the body.

Similar to the orange, the tangerine is from the orient. A healing fruit, few foods are as high in vitamin A as the tangerine.

Good for a snack and can easily take the place of sweets, there are a variety of uses for the tangerine, as in salads and vegetable dishes.

Remember, the tangerine is considered a delicate fruit. This fruit provides the body with the normal minerals and an essential vitamin for the body's skin too. Vitamin A will help provide the resistance that is needed by the body to prevent a wide variety of infections.

The reproductive organs of the body, the kidneys and the bladder, maintain good health through Vitamin A. A lack of Vitamin A in the body is often reflected through bad skin.

89

Tofu

Minerals: Calcium, Iron
Vitamins: B-Complex

Tofu is good for the body. What is Tofu? Tofu is a soft cheese-like food.

Tofu is very high in protein. A food that is low in saturated fat, tofu helps lower your blood cholesterol level. Tofu has a variety of uses and replaces the use of cheese in many dishes.

Tofu and soy (as in soybean crops) are eaten every single day by the Africans and Japanese, the world's longest living human beings. Tofu is not a natural food as is vegetables and fruits, but it does provide the body with essential minerals and vitamins for good health.

Tofu has an impressive nutritious value. High in protein as well as iron and calcium, tofu can be used to completely replace the taste of cheese in food menus and food dishes.

90

Tomatoes

Minerals: Potassium
Vitamins: A, C

Fresh tomatoes can be eaten by themselves. Tomatoes are good for your heart and they do help prevent cancer.

Rich in Vitamins A and C, tomatoes contain the amount of potassium that is necessary to help fight heart disease.

Tomatoes are plants that can grow just about anywhere there is a fertile well-drained soil. Supermarkets are generally supplied with tomatoes the year round. Tomatoes are so widely used today, they are grown in numerous mechanized systems to harvest and process them abundantly and repeatedly. Very fresh tomatoes can be grown on your own, in your own yard, garden or in the home.

The flavor of tomatoes do not vary very much, tomatoes are most commonly known in the use of ketchup, a widely used food.

Tomatoes are a healthy fruit that should be truly enjoyed.

91

Trout

Minerals: Phosphorus, Calcium
Vitamin: A, B-3 (Niacin)

The trout is an extremely nourishing food. Fish do provide needed amino acid to the body that is essential to good health.

As a sea food, trout is a seasonal fish. When foods that are eaten for good health are out of season, then a substitute must be considered during the off-season. Fish oil and cod-liver oil from this fish helps prevent cancer and other diseases in the body.

Trout as an edible fish for meat and known as poultry, come in a wide variety of types. As a choice for meat, the use of fish in particular can be considered a healthy choice. Fish do digest quicker than most widely eaten meats. The nutritional value of trout can also be a reason to strongly consider fish as a source for protein. The cold waters where the trout lives, as fresh water fish, will help guarantee a clean and fresh food.

92

Tuna

Minerals: Phosphorus, Calcium
Vitamins: A

Tuna is high in phosphorus. Essential in the normal formation of the teeth and bones, phosphorus is necessary to maintain the health of bones for the rest of your life.

Tuna is a meaty fish that is best eaten when fresh. Tuna is often canned. Used in a variety of dishes, tuna is one of the most widely distributed fish throughout the world.

Fish oil which is found in tuna is one of the healthiest of fatty acids offered to the body as the omega-3, essential to help strengthen the body's cell membranes and to help prevent cancer. The fish oil also aids in the thinning of blood in the body, which help prevent clogged arteries. Another healing aspect of this same fish-oil and as cod-liver oil, is, it helps relieve rheumatoid arthritis, which includes swelling and stiffness.

93

Turnips

Minerals: Iron, Calcium
Vitamins: A, B, C

The turnip is considered a herb. It is well known for its edible root. The most popular, turnip green is a widely eaten vegetable.

Turnips help prevent cancer. A round two inch white and firm circular or spindle-shaped root, the turnip is an excellent Vitamin B food.

The B-Vitamins are essential for the proper function of the nervous system. Included in the B-Vitamins are, B-1, B-2, B-6, B-12 that also includes folic acid.

Thiamine is included in Vitamin B-1. When the body lacks B-1, muscular weakness occurs as well as many other commonly known ailments such as leg cramps or serious heart failure. Another B-Vitamin, B-2 is Riboflavin. Riboflavin serves as a coenzyme to combine with others for effective operation in metabolism of carbohydrates and fats.

B-Vitamins are found in many natural foods, including leafy green vegetables and many grain foods.

94

Vegetables

Vegetables heal the body through the variety of minerals and vitamins that are available in their original state as a natural foods.

A nutritious food for the body, the green leafy vegetables are highly credited with the B-Vitamins, often overlooked as one of the best sources of providing needed nutrition for the body.

Thiamine found in B-1, riboflavin in B-2, niacin in B-3, pyridoxine in B-6 and cobalamin in B-12 can often be overlooked when they are not know for the importance of the vitamins they contain. Other B-Vitamins such as biotin, and folic acid plays an important role in the good health of the body.

Treatment for ailments and the healing process of damaged parts to the body require the intake of a variety of vitamins including the B-Vitamins.

Vegetables do provide a very important source of the most important nutrients the overall body needs. Many of those most important vegetables for the body are mentioned as a part of this study.

95

Walnuts

Minerals: Iron, Magnesium
Vitamins: B-1 (Thiamine)

Walnuts are widely grown throughout the world. A fruit that offer the body minerals that are not found in all foods, magnesium is needed to give the body a balance that can often be overlooked.

The walnut is well known as a tree. Walnut furniture is directly derived from the timber of the tree. The fruit that grows on the walnut tree, the tasty hard shelled nut inside, is a edible meat that is a chewy source of a needed healing mechanism for the human body.

Magnesium can lower the risk of heart disease and help prevent a stroke from occurring to the body.

Walnuts may not be easily digested, for many people, it is their natural state as a food that makes them a source for the body's health process to be maintained and restored.

96

Watermelons

Minerals: Sodium, Iron, Silicon
Vitamins: A, C

Watermelon is highly recommended as a sweet fruit. A popular desert in many cafeterias, watermelon do offer the body minerals that are an absolute necessity, for the body.

Silicon, found in the watermelon, also aids the skin, the bones and the teeth. It has been known for years that silicon fights the development of tuberculosis in the body.

There are two distinct and common flavors of the internal flesh that most people are familiar with, the red and yellow. Often called meat, watermelons are generally sweet and extremely watery.

Many deserts can be too harmful to the body when sweeten, with refined sugar, however, the watermelon a natural fruit, sweet and crisp, can help improve the health of those that must satisfy a sweet taste.

97

Wheat Germ

Minerals: Phosphorus, Calcium
Vitamins: A

Wheat germ is a widely used health food. The natural wheat itself has been cultivated to be an edible grain that can be applied to food in a variety of ways.

It is the high fiber along with the minerals and vitamins the body receive that have made wheat germ a popular food to be eaten directly.

Wheat is one of the most valuable crops grown throughout the world. We are most familiar with wheat in cereal and bread. Wheat is very high in protein, an essential need of the body.

Wheat germ can be purchased in the supermarket? Wheat germ is added to many drinks for breakfast and even included in small quantities in all types of edible dishes.

98

Yams (sweet potato)

Minerals: Phosphorus, Calcium
Vitamins: A, C

If you want to reduce your chances of lung cancer, eat sweet potatoes. Sweet potatoes, known as yams, are very high in Vitamin A. They can help prevent lung cancer. Not the Vitamin A alone, but the carotene that is in the sweet potato, will help prevent lung cancer.

Sweet potatoes are widely known. The sweet potato pie is one of the most common desserts made from the sweet potato.

There are a variety of ways to serve the sweet potato. It can be baked and eaten. Many people make candied yams from the sweet potato.

The sweet potato is a herb. Herbs are plants that specifically provide an aid to healing the human body. High in Vitamin A, this is the primary vitamin that aids the mucus membrane. A deficiency in Vitamin A help contribute to ailments such as sinuses and other irritating affects to the body.

99

Yeast (brewers)

Minerals: Phosphorus, Calcium, Iron
Vitamins: B-2 (riboflavin)

Very high in protein, brewers yeast can be a life saver. Brewers yeast is used in cooking and in beverages.

An excellent source of minerals, protein and vitamins B-Complex, brewers yeast is higher in helping prevent diseases than any other source of protein.

Yeast is widely used throughout the world. Originally yeast is most common in making bread. Many beverages use yeast in their fermentation process.

The medical connection to brewers yeast are known for their source of thiamine and B-Complex to help heal the human body.

Yeast is most commonly known in the bread making and brewing process because of its ability to ferment.

100

Yogurt

Minerals: Protein, Calcium, Magnesium, Iron
Vitamins: A, C, D

Yogurt is a dairy product. A food high in protein and calcium, this is a definite healer for the human body. Yogurt will help the body to produce vitamins the body needs. Primarily good for the intestinal track, yogurt provides the bacteria needed to ward-off infections that can develop inside the intestine and cause cancer.

The Vitamin D is the sunshine vitamin, needed for the health of the body's skin, which is also in yogurt.

Other dairy products, such as milk do offer the body high amounts of Vitamin D. Large quantities of vitamins or minerals, too often, can be harmful to the body. Eaten in moderation, foods containing needed nutrients for the body, as yogurt, do help heal the body and maintain good health.

A Gram of Prevention

Many people do jump to the eager conclusion that there are foods they do not like, when it comes to natural foods, such as fruits and vegetables.

Natural foods do give the body the needed nutrients in minerals and vitamins that protect the body against, diseases such as cancer, ailments such as allergies and even a break-down of the immune system.

The lack of knowledge causes many people to be totally unaware that most of their health problems, from poor skin to the common cold is a direct result of the lack of particular minerals or vitamins from their food intake.

The body often looses it's good protection from retained minerals and vitamins through the normal process of using them as needed, including the cleansing process of the kidneys cycle of eliminating the body's waste. Foods that provide all of the needed minerals and vitamins that the body needs, should be eaten on a regular basis. To know what foods provide for the body is each and every person's responsibility.

With the correct information on foods, you can avoid the chance of poor health suddenly taking over your body as it ages.

The Body's Organs

There are four major organs of the body that are generally infected and develop diseases. The heart, liver, lungs and kidneys are the most widely infected organs in the body.

With proper nutrition, these organs can be kept in good condition. When infections occur in the body from lack of the necessary agents inside the body to fight-off germs, serious diseases develop.

In an effort to help prevent serious infections to the major organs in the body, preventive measures can be taken by eating foods that are known to provide the necessary minerals and vitamins that protect the body.

Through eating the best foods the body needs, most any serious ailment can be prevented. When there is a desire to maintain excellent health for the body, sickness can be avoided by eating the best natural foods.

As the body receives the nutrients that are essential for good health, a protection of the vital organs will occur to help prevent the development of any serious disease. These Foods

These are not all of the foods that heal the body and provide the nutrients the body needs. This is a list of the most common foods that are easy to locate in most supermarkets. The body's energy system require these foods on a regular basis.

The body's metabolism is the process of food turning into energy. When food is digested inside the body, it is broken-down to aid the cells and tissues into rebuilding themselves. As food is digested, it separates into proteins, fats and carbohydrates in the digestive tract. The second part of the digestion process, causes proteins to split into ammonia acids, and for the carbohydrates to turn into sugar—while the blood carries them to the body's tissues, the cells uses the minerals and vitamins. Foods that cause the metabolism process to speed-up to burn excess fat is what helps the body to loose its excess. When the body continues to exhibit hunger, it can often be contributed to the lack of fiber. Foods rich in fiber help the body to register full. Many people overeat because they lack the proper fiber in their meals. This metabolism process points to the importance of proper nutrition as a way of getting all of the needed minerals and vitamins the body require to maintain good health.

What Minerals and Vitamins Really Do For The Body

Nutrients the body use to produce energy are provided through the minerals and vitamins in the foods we eat—this is what most of them do.

- **Calcium** is the bone and teeth mineral that also lowers risk of heart disease, colon cancer and high blood pressure.
- **Chlorine** from natural foods will heal the digestive system.
- **Iodine** controls metabolism and promotes growth of the body.
- **Iron** is essential for red blood cells and the immune system.
- **Magnesium** improves the nerves and maintains blood sugar.
- **Manganese** helps bone formation and muscle coordination.
- **Phosphorus** is good for longevity of the body and life itself.
- **Potassium** lowers blood pressure, improve nerve cells and muscles.
- **Protein** mends the body's tissues.
- **Silicon** helps the skin, bones and teeth to develop properly.
- **Sodium** is necessary for the human body to maintain life.
- **Sulfur** cleans the blood and adds beauty to the skin, hair and nails.
- **Zinc** helps reproduction organs and the normal healing of the body.
- **Vitamin A** helps protect the body against infections and lung cancer.
- **Vitamin B's** helps metabolism, digestion and the nervous system. **Vitamin C** protects against cancer, heart disease, lowers

blood pressure and cholesterol, while it prevent infections and heal wounds.

- **Vitamin D** helps bones and teeth formation.
- **Vitamin E** protects the cardiovascular system and prevent diseases.
- **Vitamin B-Complex** promote cell growth and reproduction.
- **Vitamin B-3 (Niacin)** will prevent fatigue, high blood pressure, nervousness, leg cramps, headaches and improve the digestive system.
- **Vitamin B-12** is good for the nervous system and body cells.

Food Sources For Minerals and Vitamins

The nutrients the body needs for restoring good health is found in the minerals that provide the body with what it needs. This is a list of good foods where those minerals can be obtained:

Calcium
- Apples
- Carrots Garlic
- Oranges
- Potatoes
- Spinach
- Tomatoes

Chlorine
- Cabbage
- Celery
- Coconut

Chlorine
- Dates
- Garlic
- Potatoes
- Tomatoes

Fluorine
- Carrots
- Celery
- Cucumbers

- Parsley
- Spinach

Iodine

- Asparagus
- Carrots
- Green peppers
- Okra
- Pineapple
- Spinach
- Turnip greens

Iron

- Almonds
- Asparagus
- Carrots
- Cucumbers
- Lettuce
- Turnips
- Tomatoes

Iron

- Avocado
- Brazil Nuts
- Cod (fish)
- Grapes
- Oranges
- Pineapple
- Raisins
- Soybean
- Strawberries
- Walnuts
- Watermelon

Magnesium
- Apples
- Bananas
- Blackberries Carrots
- Celery
- Cucumbers
- Garlic
- Lemons
- Lettuce
- Oranges
- Pecans
- Pineapple
- Tomatoes

Manganese
- Almonds
- Apples
- Carrots
- Cucumbers
- Parsley
- Walnuts

Phosphorus
- Asparagus
- Blackberries
- Brazil Nuts
- Brussels sprouts
- Cabbage
- Carrots
- Cauliflower

Phosphorus
- Garlic
- Lettuce
- Limes

- Oranges
- Potatoes
- Tomatoes
- Turnips

Potassium

- Bananas
- Carrots
- Cauliflower
- Celery
- Dates
- Garlic

Potassium

- Grapes
- Lemons
- Oranges
- Parsley
- Peaches
- Pears
- Potatoes
- Spinach
- Tomatoes
- Turnips
- Watermelons

Protein

- Almonds
- Brewer's yeast
- Brown rice
- Cottage cheese
- Lamb
- Lima beans
- Oysters
- Sunflower seeds
- Wheat germ

Silicon
- Asparagus
- Carrots
- Cucumbers
- Green peppers

Silicon
- Okra
- Pineapple
- Turnip greens
- Watermelon

Sodium
- Apples
- Carrots
- Celery
- Cucumbers
- Dates
- Grapes
- Grapefruit
- Lemons
- Lettuce

Sodium
- Oranges
- Peas
- Spinach
- Strawberries
- Tomatoes
- Watermelon

Sulfur
- Apples
- Brazil nuts
- Brussels sprouts
- Cauliflower

- Cabbage
- Garlic
- Pineapple

Zinc

- Beans
- Bread (rye)
- Chicken
- Cottage cheese
- Fish
- Lamb
- Lima beans
- Lobster
- Oatmeal
- Oysters
- Peas
- Rice (brown)
- Spinach
- Salmon
- Toufu

Zinc

- Turkey
- Whole Wheat Bread
- Wheat bread
- Yogurt

Protein

Protein is necessary for healthy cells in the body. A healthy life with vigorous activity, allowing you to reach old age is supported by a body that maintains a refreshing degree of protein. To know the list of foods that help provide needed protein when the body is lacking, and especially during the healing process, is invaluable.

Proteins are what provide the body with living substance. Proteins are combinations of the essential amino acids inside the body. Derived from food, the amino acids that combine with oxygen and other agents to form the composition of protein, provide an unlimited number of healing aids to the body. The body's cells use protein to maintain excellent health and good nutrition.

Protein provides the body with the essential amino acids that are an absolute necessity for the body to survive and live. Every individual part of the human body needs protein for normal growth and development. Protein helps the body maintain it's youthful appearance and health.

Vitamin B-Complex

The most vital vitamin to the entire body is B-Complex. The Vitamin B-Complex is primarily for keeping the human body alive. Needed for reproduction, Vitamin B-Complex comes in numbered B's. Each of these complexes of B, have a distinct meaning for the needs of the body.

Low body resistance is due to a shortage of Vitamin B-Complex. All the vitamins are needed, however, B-Complex promotes cells and living organisms. Vitamin B-Complex is what helps breaks down glucose (sugar) in the body, helping prevent the development of diabetes.

A lack of Vitamin B-Complex also causes skin problems, usually dryness, cracking, and tender skin. Even the nervous system depends on the B-Complex, B-1(Thiamine), to help promote relaxed nerves. Another of the important vitamins of the B-Complex include B-2 which offer riboflavin, known to contribute to the body's development of energy. Vitamin B-12 contain cobalt, which help cure and prevent arthritis.

Often overlooked, the Vitamin-B is what provides the body with the needed biotin and niacin that stimulate the brain and our mental health.

Foods that provide niacin to the body includes: cereal, cod fish, sardines, salmon, chicken breast and turkey breast.

Amino Acid

The amino acids combine to build protein the body needs for energy. Raw foods such as carrots, celery and cucumbers provide the high degree of amino acid the body needs.

Composed of hydrogen, oxygen, carbon and nitrogen; amino acids are contained in the following fruits and vegetables:

- Lemons
- Grapefruit
- Celery
- Apples
- Spinach
- Tomatoes
- Pineapple
- Carrots
- Beets
- Cabbage
- Garlic
- Cucumbers
- Olives
- Grapes
- Pears
- Almonds
- Raisins
- Oranges
- Lettuce
- Spinach

- Strawberries
- Okra
- Watermelon

Phosphorus and Calcium

Phosphorus and calcium are common minerals, found in many natural foods. Phosphorus is an absolute necessity for the bones and teeth. A lack of phosphorus for the body results in ailments that includes disorders of the nervous system, a body weakness and even fatigue.

Calcium through menus, help lower the risk of heart disease, and it help prevent cancer. The lack of calcium in the body can cause ailments that are commonly known as insomnia, sore muscles, and even nerve problems.

Eating natural foods provide phosphorus and calcium to the body.

Antioxidants

Foods that contain antioxidants produce the protection needed to fight diseases inside the body. Antioxidants are found in Vitamin C, Vitamin E, and Beta Carotene. There is a limit on the body's intake to prevent a toxic effect on the internal system. When toxic, poison has occurred. Too much of one chemical from foods can harm the body. An over abundance of any one food can do serious harm to the body. Eating foods in moderation that do contain antioxidants will help prevent heart disease and lung cancer.

Beta Carotene is usually found in green and yellow vegetables as well as fruits. Beta Carotene helps the skin to remain healthy. Vitamin C will help reduce wrinkles in the skin. Vitamin E will help slow the body's aging process.

Antioxidants help reduce the damage to cells inside the body—while damaged cells often do lead to the development of cancer.

Fiber

Fiber can help provide good health to the body. It will give the body the message to fill full. Eating foods with fiber will help prevent cancer in the various organs of the body. The best sources of fiber should include:

- Apples
- Barley
- Bananas
- Blueberries
- Broccoli
- Brussels sprouts
- Carrots
- Greens
- Kidney Beans
- Oatmeal
- Peas
- Pears
- Pumpkin
- Prunes
- Raisins
- Spinach
- Strawberries
- Sweet Potato (yams)
- Tomatoes

The above list represents the most common foods found in many supermarkets. These foods provide fiber to the body, which is an absolute necessity for maintaining the body's excellent health.

The Sweet Tooth

For many people, the craving for something sweet can become harmful to the body if the proper foods are overlooked. Refined sugar as used in many pastries and as a sweetener, is very harmful to the body.

To help the body improve while keeping it healthy and satisfying the sweet tooth, keeping a variety of natural foods at your fingertips can both satisfy the sweet tooth and greatly improve your health. Some of the most common natural sweet foods to consider are:

· Bananas
· Apples
· Cherries
· Grapes
· Peaches
· Raisins
· Prunes
· Oranges
· Pineapple
· Blackberries
· Cantaloupe
· Strawberries
· Watermelon
· Avocado
· Raspberries
· Nectarines
· Pears
· Mangoes

- Plums
- Tangerines

This list represents the idea that natural foods can replace many manufactured sweets which often contain harmful ingredients that can destroy the good health of the human body. Additional natural sweets are available in different regions and at seasonal times to produce specific natural foods.

Water

The blood is about three-fifths water. To clearly understand how much of the body consist of water—it takes five-fifths to obtain a complete whole, while three-fifths is more than half of that whole.

Water plays a vital role in the health of the human body. Totally separate from nutrients, water is essential for good health.

Water will dissolve the nutrients inside the body while it help carry those nutrients to the different parts of an organism. Through a chemical reaction inside the body, organisms will turn nutrients into energy. The chemical reactions that occur must take place in a watery solution inside the body. Inside the body water is needed to carry waste for organisms. The body must take-in water daily to replenish the body's normal supply of water that it needs. If the body looses more than twenty percent of it's normal water content, it will die. To maintain good health, water is essential to the daily needs of the body.

Sunlight

Sunlight can heal the body. Too much sunlight can be harmful. The rays from the sun benefit the circulation system as well as the muscles inside the body. The exposure to the sun will help the skin produce vitamin D, commonly known as the sunshine vitamin.

Much different from a sun lamp that provide only ultraviolet rays, the natural sun produce many different types of light rays useful to the human body, especially for healthy skin.

Infrared rays from the sun, penetrate very deep into the body and work as a healer. Without over exposure, sunlight is necessary to the normal health of the human body.

Exercise

Exercise is good for the health of the body, and it does not have to be strenuous. Normally, ten minutes in the morning and ten minutes in the evening would be adequate to help keep the heart in proper condition.

Walking is a great form of exercise. Even a simple one-block walk around your neighborhood, pays the heart back in a very rewarding way. The good condition of the heart, can often depend on the amount of exercise the body receives. Walking will help pump the blood more vigorously through the heart, which is a good method to keep a healthy blood circulation in the body.

Afterthought

This book will not only do wonders for you, it will help you perform miracles for your body's health, through eating foods that provide the proper nutrition for the body. *By no means is this a medical dictionary.* Many people never eat the foods their body require, they only eat what they want, which makes it easy to understand the reason people have so many ailments and why many of them are in poor health.

Inside this book is the best natural medication you could ever provide for the body. Just do your body a favor, and try them. They will improve and prolong your life, if you are in tuned to your own body's health needs.

Know when your body is in need of more nutrients and you will suddenly discover the wonders of good health. Providing the source of those needed nutrients by way of vitamins and minerals through healthy foods is what this book was intended for. Natural foods do heal the body and can provide a genuine source of the proper nutrition to help restore your body's excellent health.

The information in this book is intended to help educate people on the value foods offer on good health, not as a substitute for consultation with a physician.

About the Author

Alfred Dawson was born and raised in Atlanta, Texas. After graduation from High School, he enlisted in the U.S. Air Force as an Airman. He is a graduate of Prairie View A&M University in Texas and lives in his hometown—Atlanta, Texas.

Sources

Elwood, Cathary. *Feel Like A Million*. Pocket Books, NY. 1977

Gregory, Richard Claxton. *Dick Gregory's Natural Diet for Folks Who Eat: Cooking With Mother Nature*. Harper and Row. 1973

Hausman, Patricia and Hurley, Judith. *Healing Foods*. Dell Publishing, N.Y. 1989.

Microsoft ENCARTA Encyclopedia. Funk and Wagnalls Corporation. 1996.

The World Book Encyclopedia. Field Enterprise Educational Corporation. 1976.

www.ingramcontent.com/pod-product-compliance
Lightning Source LLC
Chambersburg PA
CBHW020238290526
45784CB00003B/1031